Table of Contents

I. Introduction

A. Overview of the book

Longevity is a term that refers to the length of life and overall health of an individual, particularly those over the age of 60. The increasing lifespan of people around the world is a testament to the advancements in medical technology and treatments. In this chapter, we will take a closer look at the factors that impact longevity and health in older adults.

Physical Health

As people age, their risk of certain health conditions such as cardiovascular disease, diabetes, and some types of cancer increases. Regular exercise and a healthy diet are essential for maintaining good health in older adults. Exercise helps to improve circulation, maintain mobility and balance, and build muscle strength. A diet rich in fruits, vegetables, whole grains, and lean proteins is also crucial for maintaining overall health.

Preventive Health Screenings

Preventive health screenings are an important aspect of maintaining good health in older adults. Regular check-ups with a doctor, along with routine screenings such as blood pressure tests, cholesterol tests, and cancer screenings, can help to detect and treat health conditions early, potentially delaying the onset of age-related health problems.

Medical Advances

Advances in medical technology and treatments have made it possible for older adults to live longer, healthier lives. New treatments and technologies have been developed to help manage chronic health conditions and improve quality of life in older adults. For example, the use of artificial joints, pacemakers, and stents has made it possible for many older adults to maintain an active lifestyle, even with age-related health problems.

Mental Health

Mental health is also an important aspect of overall health in older adults. Engaging in mentally stimulating activities, such as reading, playing games, and socializing with friends and family, can help to maintain cognitive health. Maintaining strong social connections is also essential for overall well-being in older adults.

Conclusion

In conclusion, longevity and health in older adults is a complex issue that is impacted by a variety of factors. Regular exercise, a healthy diet, preventive health screenings, medical advances, and maintaining mental health and social connections are all important aspects of maintaining good health in older adults. By taking an active approach to their health, older adults can potentially improve their quality of life and live longer, healthier lives.

B. Importance of maintaining health and longevity after 60

As people reach the age of 60, their bodies undergo a series of changes that can impact their overall health and longevity. However, maintaining good health after 60 is crucial to ensure that people can continue to live fulfilling and independent lives. Here are some reasons why it's important to focus on health and longevity after 60:

1. Reduced risk of chronic diseases: Maintaining good health after 60 helps reduce the risk of chronic diseases such as heart disease, diabetes, and arthritis. These diseases can be debilitating and significantly impact a person's quality of life, so preventing them is key.
2. Improved mental health: Good physical health is closely linked to good mental health, and the reverse is also true. Maintaining good health after 60 can help reduce the risk of depression, anxiety, and cognitive decline.
3. Better mobility: As people age, they may experience a decline in mobility and dexterity. Maintaining good health after 60 can help slow this decline and ensure that people remain active and independent.
4. Increased lifespan: A healthy lifestyle can help increase lifespan, allowing people to enjoy more years of good health and happiness.

To maintain good health and longevity after 60, it's important to focus on a few key areas:

1. Diet: A healthy diet is essential to maintaining good health after 60. This should include plenty of fruits, vegetables, whole grains, lean protein, and healthy fats.
2. Exercise: Regular physical activity is crucial for maintaining good health after 60. This can include activities such as walking, swimming, and cycling, as well as resistance training to help maintain muscle mass.
3. Sleep: Getting enough sleep is important for overall health and well-being, and this is especially true after 60. Aim for 7-9 hours of sleep per night.
4. Social engagement: Maintaining social connections is important for both physical and mental health. Engage in activities with friends and family, or consider joining a local community group.

In conclusion, maintaining good health and longevity after 60 is important for leading a fulfilling and independent life. By focusing on diet, exercise, sleep, and social engagement, people can ensure that they continue to enjoy good health as they age.

II. Physical Health

A. Exercise and Physical Activity

1. Importance of exercise for older adults

As people age, they may experience a decline in physical function and an increased risk of chronic diseases. However, regular physical activity can help maintain physical and cognitive function, reduce the risk of chronic diseases, and improve overall health and well-being in older adults. Here are some reasons why exercise is important for older adults:

1. Improved physical function: Regular physical activity can help improve balance, flexibility, strength, and mobility in older adults. This can reduce the risk of falls and increase independence.
2. Reduced risk of chronic diseases: Exercise can help reduce the risk of chronic diseases such as heart disease, diabetes, and arthritis. It can also help control the symptoms of these conditions.
3. Improved mental health: Exercise has been shown to have a positive impact on mental health in older adults, reducing symptoms of depression and anxiety and improving cognitive function.
4. Increased lifespan: Regular physical activity has been linked to an increased lifespan in older adults, allowing them to enjoy more years of good health and well-being.

To reap the benefits of exercise, older adults should aim for at least 150 minutes of moderate-intensity aerobic activity per week, along with two days of strength training per week. Some examples of moderate-intensity aerobic activities include brisk walking, cycling, and swimming, while strength training can be achieved through activities such as weightlifting or resistance band exercises.

It's important for older adults to consult with a healthcare provider before starting a new exercise program, especially if they have any underlying health conditions. A healthcare provider can help develop a safe and effective exercise program that is tailored to a person's needs and abilities.

In conclusion, exercise is important for maintaining physical and cognitive function, reducing the risk of chronic diseases, and improving overall health and well-being in older adults. By incorporating regular physical activity into their daily routines, older adults can ensure that they continue to enjoy good health and independence as they age.

2. Types of exercise recommended for seniors

As people age, they may experience a decline in physical function and an increased risk of chronic diseases. Regular physical activity can help maintain physical and cognitive function, reduce the risk of chronic diseases, and improve overall health and well-being in seniors. Here are some types of exercise that are recommended for seniors:

1. Aerobic exercise: Aerobic exercise, such as brisk walking, cycling, or swimming, can help improve cardiovascular health, reduce the risk of chronic diseases, and improve overall physical function in seniors. Aim for at least 150 minutes of moderate-intensity aerobic activity per week.
2. Strength training: Strength training, such as weightlifting or resistance band exercises, can help maintain muscle mass and improve physical function in seniors. Aim for two days of strength training per week.
3. Balance and flexibility exercises: Balance and flexibility exercises, such as yoga or tai chi, can help reduce the risk of falls and improve mobility in seniors. These exercises can also improve posture and coordination.
4. Mind-body exercise: Mind-body exercises, such as meditation or tai chi, can help reduce stress and improve cognitive function in seniors. These exercises can also help improve mental health.

It's important for seniors to consult with a healthcare provider before starting a new exercise program, especially if they have any underlying health conditions. A healthcare provider can help develop a safe and effective exercise program that is tailored to a person's needs and abilities.

In conclusion, there are a variety of types of exercise that are recommended for seniors, including aerobic exercise, strength training, balance and flexibility exercises, and mind-body exercises. By incorporating a mix of these exercises into their daily routines, seniors can maintain physical and cognitive function, reduce the risk of chronic diseases, and improve overall health and well-being as they age.

3. Tips for starting and maintaining an exercise routine

Starting an exercise routine can be challenging, especially if you haven't been physically active for a while. However, with a few simple tips, it can be easier to start and maintain an exercise routine that is safe, effective, and enjoyable. Here are some tips for starting and maintaining an exercise routine:

1. Consult with a healthcare provider: Before starting an exercise routine, it's important to consult with a healthcare provider, especially if you have any underlying health conditions. A healthcare provider can help you develop a safe and effective exercise program that is tailored to your needs and abilities.
2. Set achievable goals: Set achievable goals for yourself and make a plan for how you will reach those goals. This will help you stay motivated and on track with your exercise routine.
3. Start slow and gradually increase intensity: When starting an exercise routine, it's important to start slow and gradually increase the intensity of your workouts. This will help prevent injury and ensure that you are able to progress safely.
4. Find activities you enjoy: Find activities that you enjoy, such as walking, cycling, or swimming, and make these a regular part of your exercise routine. Doing activities that you enjoy will make it easier to stick to your routine and stay motivated.
5. Make exercise a habit: Make exercise a habit by doing it at the same time every day or every other day. This will help make exercise a routine part of your life and make it easier to stick to your routine.
6. Find a workout partner: Find a workout partner to exercise with, such as a friend or a family member. Exercising with a partner can be a great way to stay motivated and hold each other accountable.
7. Mix it up: Mix up your exercise routine to avoid boredom and keep it interesting. Try different activities, such as yoga, tai chi, or weightlifting, to keep your workout routine varied and engaging.

In conclusion, starting and maintaining an exercise routine can be challenging, but with a few simple tips, it can be easier to make exercise a regular part of your life. By setting achievable goals, starting slow, finding activities you enjoy, making exercise a habit, finding a workout partner, and mixing it up, you can ensure that your exercise routine is safe, effective, and enjoyable.

B. Nutrition and Diet

1. Recommended dietary guidelines for older adults

As people age, their nutritional needs change and they may be at increased risk of chronic diseases, such as heart disease, diabetes, and certain types of cancer. A balanced and nutritious diet can help maintain health and reduce the risk of chronic diseases in older adults. Here are some recommended dietary guidelines for older adults:

1. Emphasize nutrient-dense foods: Older adults should emphasize nutrient-dense foods, such as fruits, vegetables, whole grains, and lean proteins in their diets. These foods are high in nutrients, such as vitamins, minerals, and fiber, and can help maintain overall health and reduce the risk of chronic diseases.
2. Stay hydrated: Older adults should stay hydrated by drinking plenty of water and limiting their intake of sugary drinks, such as soda and fruit juice. Staying hydrated can help maintain physical and cognitive function and reduce the risk of chronic diseases.
3. Limit saturated and trans fats: Older adults should limit their intake of saturated and trans fats, which are found in high-fat animal products and processed foods, such as fast food and baked goods. Saturated and trans fats can increase the risk of heart disease and stroke.
4. Limit sodium intake: Older adults should limit their intake of sodium, which is found in high amounts in processed foods and added to many prepared foods. High sodium intake can increase the risk of high blood pressure and heart disease.
5. Get adequate calcium and vitamin D: Older adults should aim to get adequate calcium and vitamin D in their diets, which are important for maintaining bone health and reducing the risk of osteoporosis. Good sources of calcium and vitamin D include dairy products, fortified foods, and supplements.
6. Consider supplements: Older adults may need to consider taking supplements, such as a multivitamin, to ensure that they are getting all of the nutrients they need. A healthcare provider can help determine if a supplement is needed and what type of supplement is best.

In conclusion, there are several recommended dietary guidelines for older adults, including emphasizing nutrient-dense foods, staying hydrated, limiting saturated and trans fats, limiting sodium intake, getting adequate calcium and vitamin D, and considering supplements. By following these guidelines, older adults can maintain their health and reduce the risk of chronic diseases as they age.

2. Tips for maintaining a healthy diet

Eating a balanced and nutritious diet is important for maintaining overall health and reducing the risk of chronic diseases. However, making changes to your diet can be challenging, especially if you are used to eating certain foods. Here are some tips for maintaining a healthy diet:

1. Plan your meals: Plan your meals in advance to ensure that you are eating a balanced and nutritious diet. Consider planning meals for the week on the weekend and grocery shopping accordingly.
2. Make healthy food choices: Make healthy food choices by emphasizing nutrient-dense foods, such as fruits, vegetables, whole grains, lean proteins, and low-fat dairy products. These foods are high in nutrients, such as vitamins, minerals, and fiber, and can help maintain overall health and reduce the risk of chronic diseases.
3. Control portion sizes: Control portion sizes to help maintain a healthy weight. Use smaller plates and bowls and avoid second helpings to keep portion sizes in check.
4. Cook at home: Cook at home as often as possible to have greater control over the ingredients in your meals and to limit your exposure to unhealthy foods.
5. Limit processed foods: Limit your intake of processed foods, such as fast food and baked goods, which are often high in calories, saturated and trans fats, and sodium.
6. Read food labels: Read food labels to better understand the nutritional content of the foods you are eating. Look for foods that are high in nutrients, such as vitamins, minerals, and fiber, and low in calories, saturated and trans fats, and sodium.
7. Stay hydrated: Stay hydrated by drinking plenty of water and limiting your intake of sugary drinks, such as soda and fruit juice.

8. Enjoy your food: Enjoy your food by taking your time to eat, savoring each bite, and eating mindfully. This can help prevent overeating and ensure that you are enjoying your food to the fullest.

In conclusion, maintaining a healthy diet requires planning, making healthy food choices, controlling portion sizes, cooking at home, limiting processed foods, reading food labels, staying hydrated, and enjoying your food. By following these tips, you can ensure that you are eating a balanced and nutritious diet that helps maintain your overall health and reduces the risk of chronic diseases.

3. Common nutrient deficiencies in older adults and how to prevent them

As people age, their nutritional needs change, and they may be at increased risk of certain nutrient deficiencies. These deficiencies can have a negative impact on overall health and increase the risk of chronic diseases. Here are some common nutrient deficiencies in older adults and how to prevent them:

1. Vitamin B12: Older adults are at increased risk of vitamin B12 deficiency, which can cause anemia, nerve damage, and memory loss. Good sources of vitamin B12 include meat, poultry, fish, eggs, and dairy products. Older adults who follow a vegetarian or vegan diet may need to take a vitamin B12 supplement.
2. Vitamin D: Older adults are at increased risk of vitamin D deficiency, which can cause osteoporosis, falls, and fractures. Good sources of vitamin D include sunlight, fatty fish, and fortified foods, such as milk and orange juice. Older adults who do not get enough vitamin D from their diet may need to take a vitamin D supplement.
3. Calcium: Older adults are at increased risk of calcium deficiency, which can cause osteoporosis and fractures. Good sources of calcium include dairy products, leafy green vegetables, and fortified foods, such as orange juice and tofu. Older adults who do not get enough calcium from their diet may need to take a calcium supplement.
4. Fiber: Older adults may be at increased risk of fiber deficiency, which can cause constipation, digestive problems, and an increased risk of chronic diseases, such as heart disease and diabetes. Good sources of fiber include fruits, vegetables, whole grains, and legumes.

5. Protein: Older adults may be at increased risk of protein deficiency, which can cause muscle loss, weakness, and decreased immunity. Good sources of protein include meat, poultry, fish, eggs, dairy products, and plant-based proteins, such as beans, nuts, and seeds.
6. Iron: Older adults may be at increased risk of iron deficiency, which can cause anemia, fatigue, and decreased immunity. Good sources of iron include meat, poultry, fish, leafy green vegetables, and fortified cereals.

In conclusion, there are several common nutrient deficiencies in older adults, including vitamin B12, vitamin D, calcium, fiber, protein, and iron. By eating a balanced and nutritious diet that includes a variety of nutrient-dense foods, older adults can help prevent these deficiencies and maintain their overall health. If necessary, older adults may also need to take supplements to ensure that they are getting all of the nutrients they need.

C. Sleep and Rest

1. The importance of sleep for older adults

Getting enough quality sleep is essential for maintaining overall health and well-being. As people age, their sleep patterns may change, and they may experience sleep disturbances, such as difficulty falling asleep or staying asleep. Here is why sleep is important for older adults:

1. Improves physical health: Sleep helps to restore and rejuvenate the body, reducing the risk of chronic diseases, such as heart disease, diabetes, and obesity. It also helps to boost the immune system and maintain overall physical health.
2. Enhances mental and emotional well-being: Sleep is essential for maintaining good mental health and emotional well-being. It helps to reduce stress, improve mood, and boost cognitive function.
3. Promotes longevity: Getting enough quality sleep is essential for promoting longevity. Lack of sleep has been linked to an increased risk of premature death.

4. Reduces the risk of falls: Sleep disturbances can increase the risk of falls, especially in older adults. Getting enough quality sleep helps to improve balance and coordination, reducing the risk of falls.
5. Improves memory and learning: Sleep helps to consolidate memories and improve learning. It also helps to boost cognitive function, reducing the risk of dementia and Alzheimer's disease.

In conclusion, sleep is essential for maintaining overall health and well-being in older adults. It helps to improve physical health, enhance mental and emotional well-being, promote longevity, reduce the risk of falls, and improve memory and learning. By getting enough quality sleep, older adults can help ensure that they are able to maintain their health and independence as they age.

2. Tips for improving sleep quality

Getting enough quality sleep is essential for maintaining overall health and well-being. Here are some tips for improving sleep quality:

1. Establish a regular sleep schedule: Going to bed and waking up at the same time every day can help regulate the body's natural sleep-wake cycle.
2. Create a sleep-conducive environment: Make sure your bedroom is cool, dark, and quiet. Consider using a noise machine or eye mask if necessary.
3. Limit exposure to screens: The blue light emitted by screens can interfere with sleep. Try to limit screen time before bed, and consider using blue light blocking glasses.
4. Avoid stimulants: Caffeine, nicotine, and alcohol can interfere with sleep. Try to avoid these substances, especially in the hours leading up to bedtime.
5. Exercise regularly: Regular physical activity can improve sleep quality and help you fall asleep faster. However, avoid strenuous exercise close to bedtime.
6. Relax before bed: Engaging in relaxing activities, such as reading, meditation, or taking a warm bath, can help prepare the body for sleep.
7. Limit naps: Napping during the day can interfere with nighttime sleep. If you need a nap, try to limit it to no more than 30 minutes and avoid napping in the late afternoon.

8. Avoid clock-watching: Constantly checking the clock can create anxiety and stress, making it more difficult to fall asleep. Try to avoid looking at the clock, or consider putting it in a drawer or across the room.
9. Address underlying sleep disorders: If you are experiencing persistent sleep problems, it may be due to an underlying sleep disorder, such as sleep apnea, insomnia, or restless leg syndrome. Consider speaking with a doctor or sleep specialist to address any underlying issues.

In conclusion, there are many ways to improve sleep quality, including establishing a regular sleep schedule, creating a sleep-conducive environment, limiting exposure to screens, avoiding stimulants, exercising regularly, relaxing before bed, limiting naps, avoiding clock-watching, and addressing underlying sleep disorders. By following these tips, older adults can help ensure that they are getting the quality sleep they need to maintain their health and well-being.

3. Common sleep disorders in older adults and how to address them

As people age, they may experience changes in their sleep patterns and quality. Here are some common sleep disorders in older adults and tips for addressing them:

1. Insomnia: Insomnia is difficulty falling asleep or staying asleep. To address insomnia, consider practicing good sleep hygiene, such as establishing a regular sleep schedule and creating a sleep-conducive environment. If symptoms persist, consider speaking with a doctor or sleep specialist.
2. Sleep apnea: Sleep apnea is a sleep disorder in which breathing stops and starts during sleep. To address sleep apnea, consider making lifestyle changes, such as losing weight and avoiding alcohol and sedatives. In severe cases, a doctor may recommend using a continuous positive airway pressure (CPAP) machine.
3. Restless leg syndrome (RLS): Restless leg syndrome is a sleep disorder characterized by an irresistible urge to move the legs while trying to fall asleep. To address RLS, consider making lifestyle changes, such as avoiding caffeine and alcohol. A doctor may also prescribe medications to relieve symptoms.
4. Narcolepsy: Narcolepsy is a sleep disorder characterized by excessive daytime sleepiness and sudden, uncontrollable episodes of sleep. To address narcolepsy, a doctor may prescribe medications to improve wakefulness and regulate sleep patterns.

5. REM sleep behavior disorder (RBD): REM sleep behavior disorder is a sleep disorder in which people act out their dreams during REM sleep. To address RBD, a doctor may prescribe medications to reduce the frequency and severity of episodes.

In conclusion, sleep disorders are common in older adults, and can have a significant impact on health and well-being. To address sleep disorders, consider practicing good sleep hygiene, making lifestyle changes, and speaking with a doctor or sleep specialist. By addressing sleep disorders, older adults can help ensure that they are getting the quality sleep they need to maintain their health and well-being.

III. Mental and Emotional Health

A. Cognitive Health

1. The importance of cognitive health for older adults

Cognitive health refers to the ability to think, learn, and remember. As people age, it is common for cognitive abilities to decline. However, there are many ways to maintain and improve cognitive health. Here are some reasons why cognitive health is important for older adults:

1. Maintaining independence: Good cognitive health is essential for maintaining independence and quality of life as we age. It allows us to perform daily tasks and make important decisions.
2. Reducing the risk of dementia: Maintaining cognitive health can help reduce the risk of developing dementia, such as Alzheimer's disease. Studies have shown that lifestyle factors, such as exercise, diet, and intellectual stimulation, can help reduce the risk of cognitive decline.
3. Enhancing quality of life: Good cognitive health can improve overall quality of life, allowing us to enjoy meaningful relationships, engage in hobbies, and continue learning.
4. Improving mental well-being: Good cognitive health can improve mental well-being, reducing the risk of depression and anxiety.

So, what can older adults do to maintain and improve cognitive health? Here are some tips:

1. Exercise regularly: Exercise has been shown to improve cognitive function and reduce the risk of cognitive decline. Aim for at least 30 minutes of moderate-intensity physical activity on most days.
2. Eat a healthy diet: A diet rich in fruits, vegetables, whole grains, and omega-3 fatty acids has been shown to benefit cognitive health.
3. Engage in intellectual stimulation: Engaging in mentally stimulating activities, such as reading, playing games, or learning a new skill, can help improve cognitive function.

4. Stay socially active: Social engagement has been shown to benefit cognitive health. Try to maintain relationships with family and friends, and consider volunteering or joining a social group.
5. Manage stress: Chronic stress has been shown to have negative effects on cognitive health. Try to manage stress through relaxation techniques, such as deep breathing, meditation, or yoga.

In conclusion, cognitive health is an important aspect of health and well-being, especially as we age. By exercising regularly, eating a healthy diet, engaging in intellectual stimulation, staying socially active, and managing stress, older adults can help maintain and improve their cognitive health, enhancing their overall quality of life.

2. Tips for maintaining cognitive function

Maintaining cognitive function is essential for preserving mental sharpness and reducing the risk of cognitive decline as we age. Here are some tips for maintaining cognitive function:

1. Exercise regularly: Exercise has been shown to improve cognitive function and reduce the risk of cognitive decline. Aim for at least 30 minutes of moderate-intensity physical activity on most days.
2. Eat a healthy diet: A diet rich in fruits, vegetables, whole grains, and omega-3 fatty acids has been shown to benefit cognitive health.
3. Engage in intellectual stimulation: Engaging in mentally stimulating activities, such as reading, playing games, or learning a new skill, can help improve cognitive function.
4. Stay socially active: Social engagement has been shown to benefit cognitive health. Try to maintain relationships with family and friends, and consider volunteering or joining a social group.
5. Get adequate sleep: Adequate sleep is important for cognitive health. Aim for 7-9 hours of sleep each night.
6. Manage stress: Chronic stress has been shown to have negative effects on cognitive health. Try to manage stress through relaxation techniques, such as deep breathing, meditation, or yoga.

7. Challenge your brain: Engage in mentally challenging activities, such as solving puzzles, learning a new language, or trying new things, to help improve cognitive function.
8. Stay mentally active: Keeping your mind active by reading, writing, or engaging in conversation can help maintain cognitive function.
9. Maintain a positive outlook: A positive outlook and healthy social relationships have been shown to benefit cognitive health.
10. Seek help if necessary: If you are experiencing symptoms of cognitive decline, such as memory loss or difficulty with daily tasks, consider speaking with a doctor. Early detection and treatment can help slow or prevent cognitive decline.

In conclusion, maintaining cognitive function is essential for preserving mental sharpness and reducing the risk of cognitive decline. By exercising regularly, eating a healthy diet, engaging in intellectual stimulation, staying socially active, getting adequate sleep, managing stress, challenging your brain, staying mentally active, maintaining a positive outlook, and seeking help if necessary, older adults can help maintain and improve their cognitive function, enhancing their overall quality of life.

3. Common cognitive disorders in older adults and how to address them

As we age, the risk of developing cognitive disorders increases. Some of the most common cognitive disorders in older adults include:

1. Dementia: Dementia is a progressive decline in cognitive function that affects memory, language, and thinking. Symptoms may include forgetfulness, confusion, disorientation, and difficulty completing familiar tasks.
2. Alzheimer's disease: Alzheimer's disease is the most common cause of dementia in older adults. Symptoms may include memory loss, difficulty communicating, and changes in mood and behavior.
3. Mild Cognitive Impairment (MCI): MCI is a decline in cognitive function that is greater than normal age-related changes but not as severe as dementia.
4. Parkinson's disease: Parkinson's disease is a progressive disorder that affects movement and balance. It can also cause cognitive decline, including dementia.
5. Depression: Depression is a common mental health disorder in older adults that can affect cognitive function. Symptoms may include sadness, loss of interest in activities, and difficulty concentrating.

Here are some ways to address these cognitive disorders:

1. Seek medical evaluation: If you are experiencing symptoms of cognitive decline, it is important to seek medical evaluation. A doctor can determine the cause of the symptoms and recommend appropriate treatment.
2. Medications: Medications may be prescribed to manage the symptoms of cognitive disorders, such as Alzheimer's disease or Parkinson's disease.
3. Cognitive and behavioral therapies: Cognitive and behavioral therapies may be effective in treating depression and other mental health disorders.
4. Exercise: Exercise has been shown to improve cognitive function and may help manage the symptoms of cognitive disorders.
5. Diet: A healthy diet, rich in fruits, vegetables, whole grains, and omega-3 fatty acids, may help improve cognitive function and reduce the risk of cognitive decline.
6. Social engagement: Staying socially active through relationships with family and friends, volunteering, or joining a social group, can help maintain cognitive function.
7. Mental stimulation: Engaging in mentally stimulating activities, such as reading, playing games, or learning a new skill, can help improve cognitive function.

In conclusion, it is important to seek medical evaluation if you are experiencing symptoms of cognitive decline. By seeking treatment, engaging in regular exercise, eating a healthy diet, staying socially active, and participating in mentally stimulating activities, older adults can manage and improve their cognitive health, enhancing their overall quality of life.

B. Emotional Well-being

1. The importance of emotional well-being for older adults

As we age, our emotional well-being becomes increasingly important for overall health and quality of life. Here are some reasons why emotional well-being is crucial for older adults:

1. Lifestyle changes: As we age, we may experience changes in our health, relationships, and living situations that can have an impact on our emotional well-being.
2. Loss and grief: Older adults may experience the loss of loved ones, which can lead to feelings of sadness and loneliness.
3. Health concerns: Chronic health conditions, physical limitations, and changes in physical abilities can impact emotional well-being.
4. Social isolation: As we age, we may become more isolated, which can have a negative impact on our emotional well-being.

Emotional well-being is important for overall health because it can:

1. Improve physical health: Positive emotions and a sense of well-being have been shown to improve physical health by reducing stress, lowering blood pressure, and boosting the immune system.
2. Enhance quality of life: A positive outlook on life can improve satisfaction with life and overall happiness.
3. Foster healthy relationships: Good emotional well-being can help individuals form and maintain strong relationships with others.

Here are some tips for maintaining and improving emotional well-being in older adults:

1. Stay socially active: Engage in activities that promote social interaction and connection, such as volunteering, joining a club or group, or visiting with friends and family.
2. Practice self-care: Prioritize self-care by doing things you enjoy, such as hobbies, reading, or taking walks.
3. Seek professional help: If you are experiencing persistent feelings of sadness or depression, seek professional help from a mental health professional.
4. Practice mindfulness: Mindfulness and meditation can help reduce stress and promote feelings of peace and well-being.
5. Focus on gratitude: Practicing gratitude can help improve overall mood and emotional well-being by shifting focus to the positive aspects of life.

In conclusion, emotional well-being is important for older adults for overall health and quality of life. By staying socially active, practicing self-care, seeking professional help if needed, practicing mindfulness, and focusing on gratitude, older adults can improve and maintain their emotional well-being.

2. Tips for maintaining emotional well-being

Emotional well-being is crucial for overall health and quality of life, especially as we age. Here are some practical tips for maintaining emotional well-being in older adults:

1. Stay socially active: Engage in activities that promote social interaction and connection, such as volunteering, joining a club or group, or visiting with friends and family.
2. Practice self-care: Prioritize self-care by doing things you enjoy, such as hobbies, reading, or taking walks.
3. Seek professional help: If you are experiencing persistent feelings of sadness or depression, seek professional help from a mental health professional.
4. Practice mindfulness: Mindfulness and meditation can help reduce stress and promote feelings of peace and well-being.
5. Focus on gratitude: Practicing gratitude can help improve overall mood and emotional well-being by shifting focus to the positive aspects of life.
6. Get enough sleep: Getting enough quality sleep can help improve mood and reduce stress and anxiety.
7. Exercise regularly: Regular physical activity has been shown to improve mood, reduce symptoms of depression, and enhance overall emotional well-being.
8. Healthy eating: Eating a healthy, balanced diet can help improve mood, energy levels, and overall physical health.
9. Reduce stress: Find healthy ways to manage stress, such as through exercise, meditation, or hobbies.
10. Stay engaged and mentally stimulated: Engaging in mentally stimulating activities, such as learning a new skill or playing games, can help maintain cognitive function and improve overall well-being.

In conclusion, by following these tips, older adults can maintain their emotional well-being and improve their overall health and quality of life. It is important to seek professional help if needed and to prioritize self-care and healthy habits to maintain emotional well-being.

3. Common emotional disorders in older adults and how to address them

As people age, they may experience changes in emotional well-being that can impact their quality of life. Here are some common emotional disorders in older adults and ways to address them:

1. Depression: Depression is a common emotional disorder in older adults that can cause feelings of sadness, hopelessness, and loss of interest in life. To address depression, it is important to seek professional help from a mental health professional, who may prescribe medication, therapy, or a combination of both.
2. Anxiety: Anxiety can cause feelings of worry and nervousness and can be exacerbated by life changes such as retirement or the loss of a loved one. To address anxiety, it is important to seek professional help and engage in activities that reduce stress, such as exercise, mindfulness, and relaxation techniques.
3. Dementia: Dementia is a decline in cognitive function that can cause memory loss, difficulty with language, and disorientation. To address dementia, it is important to seek professional help and engage in activities that stimulate the brain, such as reading, playing games, and learning new skills.
4. Bereavement: The loss of a loved one can cause feelings of sadness, anger, and depression. To address bereavement, it is important to seek professional help and engage in activities that promote healing, such as support groups, therapy, and volunteering.
5. Isolation: Social isolation can cause feelings of loneliness, depression, and anxiety. To address isolation, it is important to engage in activities that promote social interaction and connection, such as volunteering, joining a club or group, or visiting with friends and family.

In conclusion, it is important for older adults to seek professional help if they experience persistent feelings of sadness, anxiety, or other emotional distress. Engaging in activities that promote well-being and seeking support from family, friends, and community resources can also be helpful in maintaining emotional health and well-being.

IV. Medical Care and Preventive Measures

A. Regular Check-ups and Screenings

1. Importance of regular check-ups and screenings for older adults

Regular check-ups and screenings are important for maintaining the health and well-being of older adults. Here are some reasons why:

1. Early Detection of Health Issues: Regular check-ups and screenings can help detect health issues early on, when they are often more easily treated. For example, routine screenings for conditions like colon cancer, breast cancer, and prostate cancer can help detect these diseases in their early stages, when treatment is more likely to be successful.
2. Monitoring Chronic Conditions: Older adults are more likely to have chronic conditions such as high blood pressure, diabetes, and heart disease. Regular check-ups and screenings can help monitor these conditions, adjust treatment as needed, and prevent complications.
3. Maintaining Independence: Regular check-ups and screenings can help identify issues that may impact a person's ability to live independently, such as vision or hearing loss, and allow for early intervention to maintain independence.
4. Mental Health Assessment: Regular check-ups and screenings can also include mental health assessments, which are important for detecting and addressing issues like depression and anxiety.
5. Vaccination: Older adults are at a higher risk for certain illnesses and diseases and should receive regular vaccinations to protect against these conditions.

It is recommended that older adults schedule regular check-ups and screenings with their healthcare provider to ensure their health and well-being are being monitored. Older adults should also keep a record of their health information, including past illnesses, medications, and test results, to bring to their healthcare provider during check-ups.

In conclusion, regular check-ups and screenings are an important part of maintaining the health and well-being of older adults. By detecting health issues early, monitoring chronic conditions, and promoting independence, regular check-ups and screenings can help older adults live a healthy and fulfilling life.

2. Recommended screenings for older adults

As we age, our bodies change and become more susceptible to certain illnesses and diseases. Regular screenings can help detect these conditions early on, allowing for prompt treatment and better health outcomes. Here are some recommended screenings for older adults:

1. Cancer Screenings: Older adults should undergo regular screenings for cancers such as breast, prostate, colon, and lung cancer. Screening frequency and type may vary based on personal and family history, as well as other risk factors.
2. Cardiovascular Screenings: Older adults are at increased risk for cardiovascular disease and should undergo regular screenings for high blood pressure, high cholesterol, and heart disease.
3. Diabetes Screenings: Older adults should be screened regularly for diabetes, especially if they are overweight or have a family history of the disease.
4. Vision and Hearing Screenings: Regular vision and hearing screenings can help detect and address issues that may impact a person's ability to live independently, such as vision or hearing loss.
5. Cognitive Screenings: Regular cognitive screenings can help detect issues such as dementia and Alzheimer's disease, allowing for early treatment and support.
6. Bone Density Screenings: Older adults are at increased risk for osteoporosis, and regular bone density screenings can help detect and treat this condition.
7. Vaccinations: Older adults should receive regular vaccinations to protect against illnesses and diseases, such as the flu, pneumonia, and shingles.

It is important to note that screening recommendations may vary based on individual health, lifestyle, and family history. Older adults should discuss their specific screening needs with their healthcare provider.

In conclusion, regular screenings are an important part of maintaining the health and well-being of older adults. By detecting health issues early, promoting independence, and preventing illnesses and diseases, regular screenings can help older adults live a healthy and fulfilling life.

B. Medications and Supplements

1. Common medications used by older adults

As we age, our bodies may require different medications to manage various health conditions. Older adults are often prescribed multiple medications to treat their conditions, and it's important to understand the purpose and proper usage of each medication. Here are some of the common medications used by older adults:

1. Cardiovascular Medications: Older adults with heart disease or high blood pressure may be prescribed medications such as angiotensin-converting enzyme (ACE) inhibitors, angiotensin receptor blockers (ARBs), beta-blockers, and calcium channel blockers.
2. Pain Management Medications: Older adults with chronic pain conditions may be prescribed medications such as nonsteroidal anti-inflammatory drugs (NSAIDs), acetaminophen, and opioids.
3. Antidepressants and Anti-anxiety Medications: Older adults may be prescribed medications to manage depression, anxiety, or other mental health conditions.
4. Sleep Medications: Older adults with sleep disorders may be prescribed medications such as sedatives, hypnotics, and antihistamines.
5. Cholesterol-lowering Medications: Older adults with high cholesterol levels may be prescribed medications such as statins, bile acid sequestrants, and niacin.
6. Diabetic Medications: Older adults with diabetes may be prescribed medications such as metformin, sulfonylureas, and thiazolidinediones.
7. Osteoporosis Medications: Older adults with osteoporosis may be prescribed medications such as bisphosphonates, denosumab, and teriparatide.

It is important to understand the potential side effects and interactions of each medication, and to communicate with the healthcare provider to ensure the proper usage and management of the medications.

In conclusion, older adults often require multiple medications to manage various health conditions. By understanding the purpose and proper usage of each medication, older adults can work with their healthcare providers to ensure their medications are used safely and effectively.

2. Tips for managing multiple medications

As we age, it's not uncommon to be prescribed multiple medications to manage various health conditions. However, taking multiple medications can be confusing and it can be easy to forget to take them or take them incorrectly. Here are some tips for managing multiple medications:

1. Keep a list of all medications: Write down the name, dose, and frequency of each medication, along with the reason for taking it.
2. Discuss with healthcare provider: Talk to your healthcare provider about all medications you are taking, including over-the-counter medications and supplements, to ensure there are no interactions or duplications.
3. Use a pillbox or reminder system: Use a pillbox or phone reminder system to help you remember to take your medications on time.
4. Store medications properly: Store medications in a cool, dry place and away from direct sunlight.
5. Avoid making changes without consulting a healthcare provider: Do not make changes to your medications or stop taking them without consulting a healthcare provider.
6. Be aware of side effects: Be aware of the potential side effects of each medication, and report any changes or concerns to your healthcare provider.
7. Ask questions: If you have questions about your medications, don't hesitate to ask your healthcare provider for more information.

In conclusion, managing multiple medications can be a challenge, but by following these tips, you can ensure that you are taking your medications safely and effectively. By working closely with your healthcare provider, you can ensure that your medications are working optimally to support your health and well-being.

3. Supplements commonly recommended for older adults

As we age, it's common for our bodies to have different nutritional needs. To support optimal health, older adults may benefit from taking dietary supplements in addition to eating a balanced diet. Here are some of the most commonly recommended supplements for older adults:

1. Vitamin B12: Older adults are often at risk of Vitamin B12 deficiency due to decreased production of stomach acid. Vitamin B12 helps maintain nerve cells and red blood cells.
2. Calcium and Vitamin D: Calcium is essential for maintaining strong bones and Vitamin D helps the body absorb calcium. Older adults are at higher risk of osteoporosis, so it's important to get enough calcium and Vitamin D.
3. Omega-3 Fatty Acids: Omega-3 fatty acids are important for heart health and cognitive function.
4. Vitamin C: Vitamin C supports the immune system and helps the body absorb iron from plant-based foods.
5. Magnesium: Magnesium is important for heart health, bone health, and maintaining a healthy nervous system.
6. Probiotics: Probiotics are beneficial bacteria that support gut health and the immune system.
7. Coenzyme Q10: Coenzyme Q10 is an antioxidant that supports energy production in cells and helps maintain heart health.

It's important to consult a healthcare provider before taking any new dietary supplements, as some can interact with prescription medications or have other side effects. Additionally, supplements are regulated differently than medications and the quality and purity of supplements can vary.

In conclusion, dietary supplements can be an important part of an overall healthy lifestyle for older adults. By consulting a healthcare provider and choosing high-quality supplements, older adults can support optimal health and well-being.

C. Preventive Measures

1. Importance of preventive measures for older adults

Preventive measures are essential for promoting health and well-being in older adults. By taking steps to prevent illness and injury, older adults can maintain independence and improve quality of life. Here are some of the most important preventive measures for older adults:

1. Regular Exercise: Regular physical activity can help prevent chronic conditions such as heart disease, stroke, and diabetes. Exercise can also improve balance, strength, and flexibility, reducing the risk of falls.
2. Healthy Diet: Eating a balanced diet that includes plenty of fruits, vegetables, whole grains, and lean protein can help prevent chronic conditions and support overall health.
3. Vaccinations: Vaccinations are an important tool for preventing serious infections and illnesses, including flu, pneumonia, and shingles.
4. Screenings: Regular screenings can help detect chronic conditions early, when they are most treatable. Screenings for conditions such as high blood pressure, diabetes, and cancer can save lives and improve health outcomes.
5. Fall Prevention: Falls are a common and serious problem for older adults. Taking steps to prevent falls, such as removing tripping hazards, improving lighting, and participating in balance exercises, can reduce the risk of injury.
6. Mental Health: Mental health is important for overall well-being. Older adults should take steps to maintain emotional well-being and seek help if they are experiencing emotional difficulties.
7. Medication Management: Medications can be an important part of maintaining health, but they can also have side effects or interact with other medications. Older adults should work with their healthcare providers to manage medications effectively and avoid adverse effects.

In conclusion, preventive measures are essential for promoting health and well-being in older adults. By taking steps to maintain physical, mental, and emotional health, older adults can live fulfilling and independent lives.

2. Common preventive measures for older adults

Preventive measures play a crucial role in maintaining the health and well-being of older adults. Here are some of the most common preventive measures for older adults:

1. Regular Physical Activity: Regular physical activity can help prevent chronic conditions, improve physical function, and reduce the risk of falls. Older adults should aim for at least 30 minutes of moderate-intensity physical activity on most days of the week.

2. Healthy Eating: A balanced diet that includes plenty of fruits, vegetables, whole grains, and lean protein can help prevent chronic conditions and support overall health. Older adults should also be mindful of their calorie and nutrient intake and consider taking vitamin and mineral supplements as needed.
3. Screenings: Regular screenings can help detect chronic conditions early, when they are most treatable. Common screenings for older adults include blood pressure, cholesterol, and blood glucose tests, as well as screenings for colon, breast, and prostate cancer.
4. Fall Prevention: Falls are a common and serious problem for older adults. Taking steps to prevent falls, such as removing tripping hazards, improving lighting, and participating in balance exercises, can reduce the risk of injury.
5. Vaccinations: Vaccinations are an important tool for preventing serious infections and illnesses, including flu, pneumonia, and shingles. Older adults should talk to their healthcare provider about which vaccinations are recommended for them.
6. Mental Health: Mental health is important for overall well-being. Older adults should take steps to maintain emotional well-being, such as staying connected with friends and family, participating in activities they enjoy, and seeking help if they are experiencing emotional difficulties.
7. Medication Management: Medications can be an important part of maintaining health, but they can also have side effects or interact with other medications. Older adults should work with their healthcare provider to manage medications effectively and avoid adverse effects.

In conclusion, these common preventive measures can help older adults maintain their health and well-being, and prevent chronic conditions and serious illness. By taking an active role in their own health and working with their healthcare provider, older adults can live fulfilling and independent lives.

V. Social Connections and Engagement

A. The Importance of Social Connections

1. The importance of social connections for older adults

As people age, social connections and relationships become increasingly important for their well-being and quality of life. Here are some of the reasons why social connections are important for older adults:

1. Emotional Support: Social connections provide emotional support and a sense of belonging, which can help reduce feelings of loneliness and isolation. Having supportive relationships can also improve mental health and increase feelings of self-worth and happiness.
2. Physical Health: Studies have shown that social connections can have a positive impact on physical health, reducing the risk of chronic conditions and helping to manage existing conditions. Having strong social connections can also improve immunity and reduce stress levels.
3. Cognitive Health: Research has also shown that social connections can help preserve cognitive function and reduce the risk of developing conditions such as dementia. Maintaining social connections can also keep the brain active and engaged.
4. Purpose and Meaning: Social connections can provide a sense of purpose and meaning in life, giving people a reason to get up in the morning and participate in their communities.
5. Safety and Security: Having strong social connections can provide a sense of safety and security, helping people to feel protected and cared for as they age.

Despite the many benefits of social connections, older adults may face challenges in maintaining relationships and building new ones. This can be due to factors such as decreased mobility, the loss of loved ones, or changes in living arrangements. To overcome these challenges, older adults can participate in activities that bring people together, such as community groups, clubs, and religious organizations. They can also reach out to friends and family and seek support from healthcare providers and community organizations.

In conclusion, social connections are critical for the health and well-being of older adults. By maintaining strong relationships and seeking out new connections, older adults can enjoy a more fulfilling and meaningful life.

2. Tips for maintaining social connections

Maintaining strong social connections is essential for the health and well-being of older adults. Here are some tips for maintaining and building new social connections:

1. Stay Active: Participating in activities and events that bring people together, such as community groups, clubs, and religious organizations, can help older adults meet new people and maintain existing relationships.
2. Use Technology: With advances in technology, older adults can now easily stay connected with friends and family through video chat, email, and social media. These tools can also be used to participate in virtual communities and events.
3. Volunteer: Volunteering in the community is a great way to meet new people and give back to others. Many volunteer opportunities are available for older adults, such as mentoring programs, tutoring, or assisting at local events.
4. Travel: Traveling to new places and experiencing new things can help older adults broaden their horizons and meet new people. Joining organized tours or groups can provide a built-in social network and help reduce feelings of loneliness or isolation.
5. Seek Support: For older adults who may be struggling with social connections, reaching out to healthcare providers, community organizations, or support groups can be helpful. These organizations can provide resources and support for building and maintaining social connections.
6. Keep in Touch: Regularly reaching out to friends and family members can help maintain existing relationships and ensure that people remain connected. This can be as simple as making a phone call, sending an email, or sending a card.

In conclusion, maintaining strong social connections is important for the health and well-being of older adults. By participating in activities, using technology, volunteering, traveling, seeking support, and keeping in touch, older adults can build and maintain the social connections they need to live a happy and fulfilling life.

B. **Engaging in Hobbies and Activities**

1. The importance of engaging in hobbies and activities for older adults

Engaging in hobbies and activities can bring joy and purpose to the lives of older adults. Here are some reasons why hobbies and activities are important for older adults:

1. Physical Health: Participating in physical activities can help improve physical health and reduce the risk of chronic diseases. For example, gardening, dancing, and swimming can help improve mobility and balance, as well as provide a form of low-impact exercise.
2. Mental Health: Engaging in hobbies and activities can help reduce stress, anxiety, and depression, and improve overall mental health. For example, activities such as painting, knitting, and playing games can provide a creative outlet and help distract from negative thoughts and emotions.
3. Cognitive Health: Engaging in mentally stimulating activities, such as puzzles and reading, can help improve cognitive function and reduce the risk of cognitive decline.
4. Social Connection: Participating in hobbies and activities with others can help build and maintain social connections. For example, joining a dance class, choir, or bridge club can provide opportunities to meet new people and engage in social activities.
5. Purpose and Meaning: Engaging in hobbies and activities can bring a sense of purpose and meaning to life, and provide a feeling of accomplishment. For example, volunteering, mentoring, or pursuing a long-time interest can provide a sense of significance and contribute to overall well-being.

In conclusion, engaging in hobbies and activities is important for older adults, as it can improve physical health, mental health, cognitive health, social connections, and provide a sense of purpose and meaning. Encouraging older adults to explore their interests and engage in activities that bring joy and fulfillment can help enhance their quality of life.

2. Tips for finding hobbies and activities that are enjoyable and beneficial

Finding hobbies and activities that are enjoyable and beneficial can be a challenge for older adults, but it is important for overall health and well-being. Here are some tips for finding hobbies and activities that are both enjoyable and beneficial:

1. Explore Interests: Reflect on past hobbies and interests and consider what you enjoyed doing before. Try to rekindle old interests or explore new ones.
2. Get Active: Engage in physical activities that are low-impact, such as walking, gardening, or swimming. Participating in physical activities can improve physical health and reduce the risk of chronic diseases.
3. Try Something New: Take a class, learn a new skill or try a new hobby that you've never done before. This can be a great way to expand your horizons and challenge yourself.
4. Get Creative: Engage in creative activities, such as painting, writing, or crafting, which can provide a sense of accomplishment and improve mental well-being.
5. Join a Group: Joining a group, such as a dance class, choir, or club, can provide opportunities for social connections and engagement with others.
6. Volunteer: Volunteering for a cause you are passionate about can provide a sense of purpose and meaning and help improve mental health.
7. Seek Advice: Talk to family, friends, and healthcare providers for recommendations on hobbies and activities that may be appropriate for your health and abilities.

In conclusion, finding hobbies and activities that are enjoyable and beneficial is important for older adults. By exploring past interests, getting active, trying new things, getting creative, joining a group, volunteering, and seeking advice, older adults can find hobbies and activities that bring joy and fulfillment, while also improving physical and mental health.

VI. Conclusion

A. Summary of key points

As we age, maintaining health and longevity becomes increasingly important. Here are some key points to keep in mind for older adults to maintain a healthy and long life:

1. Exercise: Regular physical activity is essential for improving physical health, reducing the risk of chronic diseases, and maintaining cognitive function.
2. Diet: A balanced and nutrient-dense diet can help prevent nutrient deficiencies and support overall health. It is important to consume enough fruits, vegetables, whole grains, and lean protein, while limiting processed foods, added sugars, and saturated fats.
3. Sleep: Adequate and quality sleep is important for overall health and well-being. It can improve mood, cognitive function, and reduce the risk of chronic diseases.
4. Cognitive Function: Engaging in mentally stimulating activities, such as reading, writing, playing games, and socializing can help maintain cognitive function and reduce the risk of dementia.
5. Emotional Well-being: Maintaining social connections, engaging in hobbies and activities, and seeking support for mental health concerns can help improve emotional well-being.
6. Preventive Measures: Regular check-ups, screenings, and preventive measures, such as vaccinations and flu shots, can help detect and prevent health problems early on.
7. Medications: Taking medications as directed, managing multiple medications, and seeking advice from healthcare providers can help improve overall health and well-being.

In conclusion, maintaining health and longevity after 60 requires a comprehensive approach that includes regular exercise, a balanced and nutrient-dense diet, quality sleep, engaging in mentally stimulating activities, maintaining social connections, regular check-ups, preventive measures, and properly managing medications. By following these key points, older adults can increase their chances of a healthy and long life.

B. Encouragement for older adults to take control of their health and longevity

As we age, it is natural to feel a sense of uncertainty about the future. However, it is important to remember that taking control of your health and longevity is within your power. Here are some tips and encouragement for older adults to take control of their well-being:

1. Be proactive: Regular check-ups, screenings, and preventive measures can help detect and prevent health problems early on. Don't be afraid to ask your doctor about recommended tests and screenings.
2. Adopt a healthy lifestyle: Regular exercise, a balanced and nutrient-dense diet, and quality sleep can improve overall health and reduce the risk of chronic diseases.
3. Keep your mind active: Engaging in mentally stimulating activities, such as reading, writing, playing games, and socializing, can help maintain cognitive function and reduce the risk of dementia.
4. Stay connected: Maintaining social connections and engaging in hobbies and activities can improve emotional well-being and provide a sense of purpose.
5. Take care of your medications: Properly managing medications and seeking advice from healthcare providers can help improve overall health and well-being.
6. Seek support: Don't hesitate to seek support from family, friends, or healthcare professionals if you are experiencing any mental health concerns.
7. Stay positive: A positive attitude and outlook on life can have a significant impact on overall health and well-being.

In conclusion, taking control of your health and longevity after 60 is a empowering and fulfilling experience. By following the tips outlined above, older adults can improve their chances of a healthy and long life. Remember, it's never too late to adopt healthy habits and make positive changes to your lifestyle.

C. Additional resources for further information and support.

If you are looking for further information and support on longevity and health over 60, there are numerous resources available. Here are some additional books and resources that you may find helpful:

1. Books:
- "The Blue Zones Solution: Eating and Living Like the World's Healthiest People" by Dan Buettner
- "Younger Next Year: Live Strong, Fit, and Sexy - Until You're 80 and Beyond" by Chris Crowley and Henry S. Lodge, M.D.
- "The MIND Diet: A Scientific Plan to Age Proof Your Brain and Live Longer" by Maria Moskovitz
- "The New Healthy Aging Diet: Avoid the Diseases of Aging, Improve Health and Live a Long Life" by Jack Challem
2. Websites:
- National Institute on Aging (www.nia.nih.gov)
- American Geriatrics Society (www.americangeriatrics.org)
- National Council on Aging (www.ncoa.org)
- National Institute of Neurological Disorders and Stroke (www.ninds.nih.gov)
3. Support groups:
- ElderTreks (www.eldertreks.com)
- Silver Sneakers (www.silversneakers.com)
- AARP (www.aarp.org)

Dr. David Sinclair is a leading researcher and professor of Genetics at Harvard Medical School. He has written several books on the topic of aging and longevity, including:

1. "Lifespan: Why We Age and Why We Don't Have To"
2. "The Genetic Convergence: A Pioneering Program to Extend Human Potential and Longevity"
3. "The Gene Therapy Plan: Taking Control of Your Genetic Destiny with Diet and Lifestyle"
4. "The Mitochondrial Plan: A Program to Improve Your Energy, Health, and Longevity"
5. "The 2-Week Age-Reversing Plan for Health, Longevity, and Vitality"

These books offer insights into the science of aging and provide practical strategies for promoting longevity and improving health. They are written for a general audience and are accessible to readers with little to no scientific background.

Dr. Valter Longo is a researcher and professor of Gerontology and Biological Sciences at the University of Southern California. He has written several books and resources on the topic of longevity and health, including:

1. "The Longevity Diet: Discover the New Science Behind Stem Cell Activation and Regeneration to Slow Aging, Fight Disease, and Optimize Weight"
2. "The Forever Young Diet & Lifestyle: Proven Ways to Help You Stay Young and Live Longer"
3. "Fast Diet, Feast Diet: Intermittent Fasting to Live Longer and Better"
4. "The ProLon Fasting-Mimicking Diet: The Revolutionary New Way to Lose Weight and Improve Your Health by Mimicking the Effects of Fasting"
5. "Longevity Diet Video Course"
6. "The ProLon Fasting-Mimicking Diet: 5-Day Fasting-Mimicking Diet Kit"
7. "Longevity Nutri-Profile: Nutritional Assessment Tool to Optimize Health and Longevity"

These resources provide an in-depth look into the science behind longevity and offer practical strategies for optimizing health and promoting longevity.

Ben Greenfield is a health and fitness expert and has published several books and resources on health, wellness, and longevity. Some of the notable books and resources by Ben Greenfield include:

1. "Beyond Training: Mastering Endurance, Health & Life"
2. "The Low Carb Athlete"
3. "The Keto Diet: The Complete Guide to a High-Fat Diet"
4. "The Low Carb Athlete Cookbook"
5. "The Intermittent Fasting Handbook"
6. "The Complete Guide to Fasting"
7. "The Low-Carb Athlete Podcast"
8. "Get-Fit Guy Podcast"
9. "Ben Greenfield Fitness" (website)
10. "The Ben Greenfield Fitness Premium Membership"

These resources provide a wealth of information and support on health and longevity, including diet, exercise, sleep, and stress management, among others.

By exploring these resources, you can gain a deeper understanding of how to improve your health and longevity after 60. Remember to always consult with your healthcare provider before making any significant changes to your lifestyle.

In conclusion, there are many books, websites, and support groups that can provide valuable information and support on longevity and health over 60. By taking advantage of these resources, older adults can take an active role in improving their health and well-being for years to come.